Near Infrared and Near Light Therapy: For Weight Loss, Arthritis, Joint Pain, Parkinson's disease, Accelerated Healing, Detoxification and Anti-Aging

Disclaimer

This information presented herein is the opinion of the author and is not meant to substitute for medical consultations and advice. Hence, do not use this book to diagnose, cure or treat any health condition or illness, if you suspect or have a medical problem contact your physician or health care provider.

TABLE OF CONTENTS

Introduction

Hi, I'm writing this book about what a lot of people have been asking me of lately which is, what is this? Why have I been sitting in front of it every day and so I am going to write about this amazing Near Infrared (NIR) and Near Light therapy and why we have been living it as a family.

To be completely honest with you, light therapy is something that I look forward to doing every single day. I feel the difference when I wake up. Personally, after 10 to 15 minutes of doing light therapy, I feel energized, charged, driven, focused, and different throughout the rest of the day.

Light therapy, also known as photobiomodulation, has become huge and successful today because there are so many researchers finding its incredible benefits which it is having on your cells, your skin and healing in general.

Although I have come across the of concept light therapy several times, but I first became interested in it because my son is dealing with eczema and I started learning all the other benefits of it. So I knew that I wanted to get one not only for him but also for my husband.

In general, it is an amazing benefit. Then you also get the side benefits of fading scars, stretch marks, evening out skin tone, boosting testosterone, boosting collagen production, as well as speeding up wound healing.

I knew I wanted to get one at home for my skin, just because I love trying out anything that has to do with making my skin better.

Secondly, for my husband, to have an accelerated healing because he actually jumped off a cliff and tore open the bottom of his foot, really bad. And honestly, it is been amazing healing on him. I wanted to try that and for my son's eczema.

So we have been doing it every night. We give our son bath and then we all make him sit in front of it without any clothes on, just so he can get the full exposure and it is actually helped him. It is just been helping his skin.

I love right before I go to bed to just sit in front of it and read. It is such a relaxing time. I noticed a difference on my skin tone because I have a lot of broken capillaries. I really like it for that.

Honestly, it is super relaxing and helps mentally. I feel a lot better after sitting in front of it and using it every day. As for my husband, he puts his foot in front of it to help stimulate the healing and cellular rejuvenation.

I wrote about in an article on “the science and benefits of NIR and light therapy” benefits ranges from skin to cellular health to fatigue to hormonal balance.

Every time you sit in front of it, I love that for my son, for myself. It does not have any side effects. It is super safe and I am sure there is going to be so much more research coming out about it and the benefits of it.

I just love that we get to do that single day in the comfort of our home.

Thank you.

History of Red and near-infrared (NIR) radiation

So I am going to discuss on the history of this amazing light therapy. I am going to write about the amazing discovery of infrared radiation there is a really cool story behind infrared radiation and how it was discovered. I am going to share that with you today. So let's start.

What is Infrared Light?

The first thing is let's discuss about what is infrared radiation? And that is basically the type of light the entire visible light that we associate with heat that is given off by an object.

The discovery of how this radiation behaves and how it was discovered historically is what I am going to write about now. So I would like to introduce you to somebody if you have never heard of him, he is a famous scientist by name William Herschel (1738 - 1822).

The picture of our Sun is a modern picture. Of course, Herschel Willaim never saw the Sun as it is in the modern picture, but he did using a high-powered telescope or satellite as we see it today. But basically he spent a great deal of time studying light from the stars with his telescope. What he did was he put filters in front of the telescope. These filters are different color filters: red filters, yellow filters and blue filters. Its function is to basically filter the light coming from the Sun. From his studies with this telescope, he realized that the red light isolated from the Sun seemed to be hotter than the other colors (he isolated them with his filters). This was not a scientific experiment this was something he was noticing, so he decided to investigate further.

Now even back in William Herschel's day, the scientists of the time were aware that sunlight was composed of a whole host of colors of the rainbow. He knew all about prisms which could do the job. So he knew that sunlight was a mixture of all the colors of the rainbow and he knew that he could take white light and split it up into the different colors: violet, indigo, blue, green, yellow, orange and red. What he wanted to do was scientifically to see if any of these colors coming from the Sun actually had a higher temperature or did they all behave the same. So he decided to set up an actual experiment to test and see if they were all the same or if any of the colors were hotter or colder than the other.

In 1800, he devised his experiment to see if the different colors of the rainbow actually had different temperatures. To do that, he took thermometers of the day and he blackened the bulbs of the end of those thermometers because black objects absorb the most energy from light. He blackened the bulb so they would absorb the sunlight the best.

So what he would do is he would put one of the thermometers in the various colors and he had the other two thermometers that would sit outside the spectrum on. In other words, where there is no color, where there is no rainbow and he would do that as controls so he could see at the same time what the color of the different shade that he was investigating was, what the temperature was, and at the same time he could see what these outside thermometers were doing just as a control.

He found conclusively that violet which is on one end of the rainbow had the coolest temperature and as he moved two thermometers up closer to red they progressively got warmer and warmer. Also, red color was the hottest color of the visible spectrum and that is what he was noticing with his telescope all those years. He just proved it with thermometers interestingly; by complete accident he had other two thermometers outside of the visible spectrum. But what he noticed was actually amazing.

What the whole point of the story is that when he placed the thermometer just outside of the red part of the spectrum, it was actually hotter than all of the other colors in the experiment and I will let that sink into you.

So he discovered by complete accident and that is what makes the story so interesting that beyond the red light of the visible spectrum that we see exists an invisible light that was hotter than all of the visible colors that he could see so he obviously thought this was a very important discovery.He actually named these invisible rays calorific rays which to me sound a little bit like calorie. This sounds a little bit like heat to me that is where the origin of that word came from. I call them calorific rays today we actually call it infrared radiation that William Herschel discovered. What Herschel did really was he totally by accident discovered infrared radiation which is an invisible part of the spectrum that we cannot see with our eyes.

In the electromagnetic spectrum now there is a part that we can see with our eyes and those are just a range of frequencies that is basically what your eyes are sensitive to. What Herschel discovered is that if you go just past red you end up in the infrared region our eyes cannot see infrared light but it is just another frequency of electromagnetic radiation that has a slightly longer wavelength or you can think of it as a lower frequency same deal.

When I say electromagnetic radiation is basically it is just a wave that travels, that has an electric field component and a magnetic field component and together they form a wave that we can at least in the visible spectrum we can sense it. We all know that we have microwave ovens and that is just another band of the electromagnetic spectrum, we have radio wave to talk to each other on the radios and then if you go to the other end of the visible spectrum; we have red light and then we have infrared; we have the violet part of the spectrum and on the other side we have ultraviolet which of course we cannot see but that is what you worry about when you get sunburned and then we have x-rays and gamma rays which are the highest frequency.

So the bottom line here is that we know that infrared and visible light is only a very small part of this entire thing that is a continuum. You know a lot of people think we have radio waves, microwaves, infrared, and ultraviolet. They also think of them as different things but really all of those different names are just different segments of all of this radiation that is really all the same stuff.

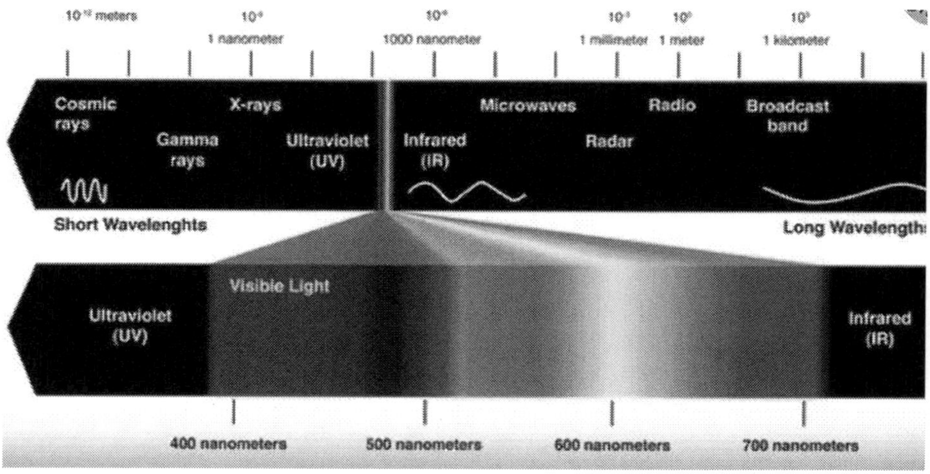

Fig. 1 Electromagnetic spectrum

Natural Sun

Natural Sun light has been used not only for growing crops but also as Helia therapy to heal the skin and cure other ailments. Modern light therapy was pioneered by Niels Finsen, a physician from the Faroe Islands. He created the first artificial light source to treat a skin infection known as "lupus vulgaris" for small pox lesions and he also used red light. In 1903, Finsen won the Nobel Prize in Physiology or medicine.

The Sun is made of various frequencies with different wavelengths. Natural sunlight consists of ultraviolet (UV) light which ranges from 300 to 400 nanometers (nm). The entire visible light spectrum is 400 to 700 nanometers and infrared light is 700 to 1200 nanometers.

Why You NEED Sunlight for Optimal Health

I want to talk about the first environmental factor that is critically important for optimal functioning and great energy in your body and that is light.Evolutionary biology and biophysics has found the mechanisms on why humans lost their fur and that was to expose our skin and also our eyes like solar panels to the Sun.

You see multiple chemical reactions occur because specific molecules are activated or inactivated by light energies. Theseinclude: hormones like melatonin, testosterone, adrenaline, cortisol, insulin and vitamins like vitamin D and neurotransmitters like dopamine and serotonin.Without going into the deep biophysics or the recent scientific discoveries we can use this information right now and put it to use to affect our help right now that is because research is confirming that what happens automatically in nature is what we need and that is before mankind changed everything by changing our light.

The Environmental Protection Agency has reported that the average American spends 93% of their time indoors, 6% of cars and 87% in buildings.That leads 7% of the time were outside and we are probably covered up we are wearing sunscreen, sunglasses hats, gloves or it's not so hardly ever in the Sun anymore.Now,just imagine you had a house that was run by solar panels on the roof and you cover them up with a coat you would get no power to the house, the food in the refrigerator or the broth and there would be no air conditioning or heat, you would not have any TV you would have no lights without power things shut down. And that is exactly what happens to a human that stays indoors and covers up from the Sun and always wear sunglasses and slathers on the sunscreen.

The Sun has a major effect on their health and it is critically important for optimal health thespecifics here will vary for each individual.It depends on your genetics, how far from the equator you live, the elevation that you live, your skin color and other factors like your climate and population density.Big cities have a lot of air pollution and so we do not get the Sun through the shade of the air pollution. New research has shown that energy flows in life are controlled by internal clocks in our brain and all other tissues.These clocks control the hundred thousand chemical reactions that occur every second in each of our 37 trillion cells.These reactions are coordinated by the internal clocks.Now the clocks for life are set to the date and night cycles of the earth and that makes sense because that is where everything evolved and that is where we live.

So if you want your energy flow to be optimal you need to get your clocks which gets the chemical reactions working in synchrony.Deep research discoveries in circadian biology show that early morning light in the eye sets the master clock which lies in the brain and the suprachiasmatic nucleus. This is caused by visible light frequencies from the Sun exciting molecules in our retina that signal the brain to set the clock.This should be a key component of addressing your environment and get your eyes exposed to the Rising Sun at this time of day.Your eyes are very sensitive to sunlight so it does not take that much to get the effect.Try to spend five minutes facing the Sun every morning even if it is cloudy because some light still penetrates into the eyes later in the day.

Another aspect of natural sunlight is that sunlight is absorbed by water in our body.Did you know that 99% of the molecules in the human body are water? When sunlight is absorbed by water, the water is charged separated which causes the body to store energy like a battery.This is a battery that gives us free energy for all kinds of duties within the body so that we can stay healthy. So just by getting in the Sun on a regular basis you can greatly improve your energy and your cellular energy.It is important not to burn yourself.

It generally takes four or five weeks of gradually increasing sun exposure for your skin to make adaptation so it can absorb more sunlight. It does this by creating melanin which absorbs light and uses that light for energy and that's a molecule that makes us tan. Also our skin thickens to make us more Sun tolerant and that's typically what happens we were outdoors in the springtime. Nature does it right.The springtime Sun gradually intensifies so when summer comes we are ready for it.We have thick tough tan skin but the bottom person is indoors and then using sunscreen so they go out in the Sun and they get burned and that damages our skin.

However, it has been shown that the body responds very positively to specific wavelengths between the 600 to 1000 nanometer ranges. This type of red and near-infrared light can pass through human tissue much more easily than other wavelengths.

You might be wondering **what is red light therapy**?

Well, scientists have basically studied light wavelengths from this spectrum to this end spectrum so a lot of white light wavelengths within that range and they have found a specific wavelength of red light to be the most beneficial for health well-being and vitality.

So what exactly is near-infrared?

Near-infrared is part of the energy Spectrum that is released from the Sun and the way I would like you to think of near-infrared as almost like a nutrient. Let me give you an example in 2016 another brand-new study released they have discovered that near-infrared when you are exposed to it in the early morning hours for a few hours (as humans were designed to do by living outside) that few hours of near-infrared in the morning had a protective factor equivalent to an SPF 15 sunscreen against the damaging ultraviolet rays that we get exposed to in the middle of the day. The study went on to show that if you then lingered in the sunlight in the evening when you were also exposed to the near-infrared that that would then help to repair the ultraviolet damage that was done during the day.

The point that I am trying to make is that near-infrared is essentially a nutrient and nature knows best and we were designed to be in it. We seem to have this great fear of sunlight and we try to get ourselves removed from sunlight but as we found out we need the Sun for certain aspects such as vitamin D production.

When red light is shined on the skin it can penetrate several millimeters into the skin where it has a beneficial biochemical effect. The mitochondria absorbed the red light which triggers our release in nitric oxide an increase in ATP production and a decrease in oxidative stress.

The science of red and near infrared (NIR) light therapy

Now the question you may be asking is how can light do all of this?

Well, it turns out that our cells contain mitochondria and that is essentially the engine of our cells and the cells that make up our tissues like muscle tissue have a particularly high concentration of mitochondria that is responsible for virtually all cellular functions such as ATP production reducing oxidative stress and even repairing muscle tissue. The term ATP production should be very familiar to you remember that supplementing with more creatine essentially supercharges the ATP to ADP back to ATP cycle to provide your muscle cells with more energy and power output.

But how is this related?

Getting back to red light therapy scientists have discovered that the mitochondria that is bountiful on your muscle tissue for instance, responds to specific wavelengths of red and infrared light with increased function. And when given the right amount of these specific wavelengths the resulting enhanced cellular function produces measurable results. One study randomly divided participants in two separate groups for an eight-week training period. One group received a red light treatment before every training session well the other group did the same training but without the light treatment. They found that the group receiving the light therapy had improvements in muscle growth 50% greater than those with muscle training alone. Amazing right? Another randomized double-blind placebo-controlled study using red and infrared light on the biceps demonstrated an average performance of more than 12% than the control group.

But while all this is very interesting I am sure you are wondering whether red light therapy is worth it and what it can do for you. First of all, I am sure many of you appreciate the science breakdown but some of you may not be able to follow along.

So here is the simple explanation, scientists have discovered that our cells show an incredible response to light but not just any kind of light only in the 660 to 1000 nanometer range which is the so called red and near infrared light range. This type of light energy penetrates deep into the skin muscle and joint tissue and stimulates the production of ATP which you should think of as your body's way of transporting energy to where it needs to go in layman's terms. More ATP means more efficient energy transfers which translates to various benefits at a cellular level. So by exposing our body to therapeutic red light our cells receive this rejuvenating anti-aging energy boost that enables them to perform every single function at a heightened level

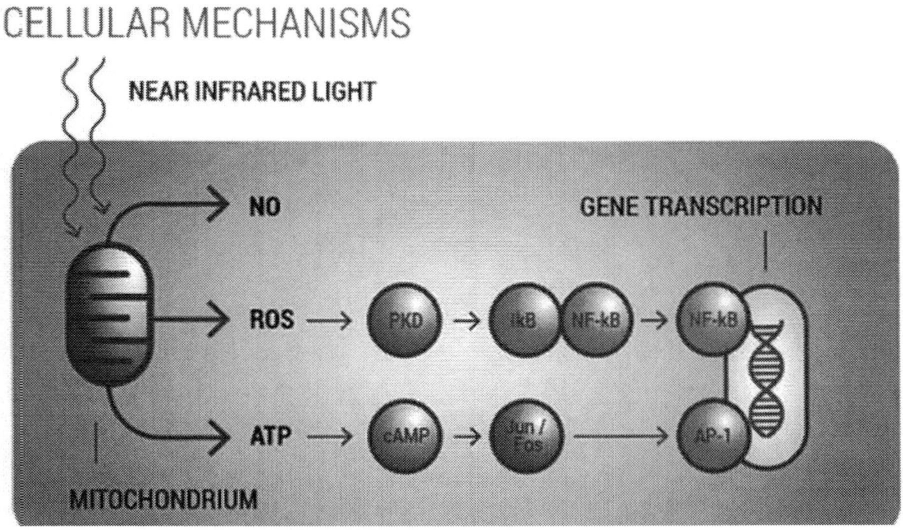

Fig. 2 Mechanisms of Near Infra-Red Light

And now that you understand the science behind it let's take a look at the four reasons why it might be a good idea for you to invest in this technology.

Number one for increased energy and testosterone:

Do you feel lethargic and out of energy a times, like your body is constantly running on empty. Then, you spend some time outside on a nice hot summer day and all of a sudden you feel amazing right? It is because our bodies rely on light as a source of energy, helping our glands to regulate adrenaline, testosterone metabolism and several other functions. And it has been shown that red light therapy can increase testosterone production for males, which in terms can increase overall energy levels and even improve peak muscle performance.

Number two for reduced muscle and recovery time:

After a challenging workout, your body is working around the clock to repair and strengthen torn muscle fibers. We know this. We also know that nutrition plays a huge role in providing the body with the resources it needs for this process but what most of you do not know is that specific wavelengths of light play a role in this process. And by enhancing mitochondrial function red light has been proven to produce measurable gains in peak strength and reduced recovery times.

Number three for faster healing for joint and muscle injuries:

Injuries, repetitive motion or aging in general can lead to severe joint pain and tissue damage but the body's natural healing response can be greatly accelerated by red and infrared light. Also, relief from pain, faster recovery times and reduced symptoms of arthritis are just a few more of the benefits of red light therapy for bodybuilders.
Yes, light is also great for reduced or delayed onset muscle soreness after all it is a type of muscle tissue injury as well.

Number four for stress relief:

You cannot argue that our mind and body is under constant stress because of the busy lives we lead. Red light therapy has been proven to calm our physical and mental state by reducing oxidative stress. I cannot personally attest to that simply because some days my stress is through the roof and other times I get my mind right and just relax but it makes sense. Oxidative stress is not just harmful to our physical health but also to our mental state as well. For me personally especially with all the traveling I have been doing lately being able to utilize red light therapy in my home has helped me stay on track with my training. It might seem silly to you but one a few things I hate about traveling is that when I get home and hit my routines hot again I get incredibly sore for the first week or two. This is because I am not able to reach the same kind of intensity that I get when I workout at home versus when I am traveling around the world. My legs get super sore after a hardcore leg work out or if I go running for like five or six miles the first time always leaves my leg sore. But after using red light therapy before and after training I can honestly say I am still sore but not as much and I am able to recover much quicker as well.

The benefits of Near Infrared and Near Light Therapy

I want to share with you information about near red light here. You know this is something that I have been doing every single morning since I got the device and I am really grateful for this technology because of the health effects and benefits that come from it.

I have been using the near infrared light therapy for months now so I thought I would do a start with the benefits itself and it is been studied all over the world so there is just a long list of proven benefits.

It helps with muscle recovery and fade scars, stretch marks and wrinkles. Also, it speeds up wound healing and decreases joint inflammation. In addition, it helps with infertility, enhances thyroid function, and men uses it to help their testosterone production.

Personally, in the six months that I have been using, it I have noticed quite a few different things. I have an overall better sense of well-being which is kind of hard to describe but it is noticeable for me and I am sleeping better. I feel like I have a little more energy, I definitely think it helps with fighting off the winter blues I am in the northern climate so any little bit that can help me get through winter is a plus for me. My skin is definitely improving, there is a glow to it which I love obviously and I think it helps me sleep better at night. My husband uses it as well and he has liked it. We have noticed a little bit less stiffness after working out. I am 30 and I do not feel like I should be feeling stiffen; you know kind of sore but I'm noticing that a little more but using near light therapy, I feel like it does help my muscles recover after workouts and I am moving a little less slowly and feeling a little less creepy so that's a really nice improvement and my husband's been enjoying that as well. Another thing I have noticed and I can't prove this but I am hoping it's a result of it, is that I have been getting sick less and currently, I am actually doing better and staying healthier.

Like I mentioned earlier, the Sun and light can be broken into different spectrums just like food can be broken into different nutrients. These different spectrums of light affect your biology and your cells differently. I would say the biggest benefit that I really like about is the findings on how near red and infrared spectrums of lights affects your mitochondria. Mitochondria are like the powerhouse of all your cells which produce (Adenosine triphosphate) ATP; the cellular energy. It benefits your energy levels by increasing the ATP molecule. Hence, it keeps your energy levels up and it improves your sleep.

Similarly, near light therapy helps to naturally stimulate tissue and rejuvenate skin through increased circulation, fibroblast stimulation, collagen production and the release of cellular energy (ATP). In other words, it improves collagen production in the skin, so if you have like fine lines and wrinkles it actually helps to heal them. If you have wounds, eczema, acne or any skin conditions it's also beneficial.

It is also beneficial for stimulating the lymphatic system which is the fluid within your body that needs to move in order for your body to detoxify itself.

It is even beneficial for seasonal affective disorder. For instance, if you live in the northern hemisphere like myself, it is beneficial for that time of the year that window period that there's not as much sunlight. That is gray outside. That is when most people are diagnosed with seasonal affective disorder which is really just a lack of sunlight; so if you live in the north and you feel a little bit down or depressed within that season or period near light therapy will be beneficial.

It is also beneficial for boosting your immunity level, for blood health circulation and lymphatic system. It is just energizing, it charges you and I think that is what I love about it. I love things that energizes me because I am a high-energy person so I use my energy to express myself or create something and I can easily just come get pooped out. So you know like I do not want to burn myself out intentionally and this is something that allows me to sustain higher levels of natural energies throughout the day. I do not drink coffee or anything like that I do not have caffeine because I found out recently that caffeine depletes essential minerals and trace minerals, as well as it depletes potassium which 98% of the population in the United States is deficient in. So if you're drinking caffeine as a source of energy, you are depleting the very mineral that gives your life the needed vitality in blood circulation, muscles and nervous system.

If you work in the corporate world or you are busy or you travel a lot this is something you need at home. Interestingly, a lot of professional sports teams or professional sports organizations or teams, athletes, people that play in the NFL and the NBA UFC fighters all these different types of use red light as part of their training routine. Hence, it is beneficial for physical recovery performance because what the red light therapy does is by increasing circulation it is allowing more nutrients and oxygen to circulate to your muscles to recover your body faster and sooner.

If you have insomnia or if you wake up in the middle of the night or if you have any of these kind of sleep related issues or energy related issues this is a something I'll definitely consider as an investment into your health because like I said it's a one-time investment it's not cheap but it's totally worth it.

In summary, the benefits of exposure to near infrared light energy include the following: reduced appearance of wrinkles; fine lines and crow's feet, improved skin tone texture and complexion, softer smoother skin and diminished pore size, increased skin elasticity and moisture retention, decreased inflammation and puffiness as well as improved hair texture and growth.

There are specific wavelengths that have been documented to have the most profound effect on enhancing cellular function. And so what specific wavelengths within that therapeutic window do is they actually break that bond between cytochrome C oxidase and nitric oxide almost releasing it to help induce normal cellular function at the core. That's why you get such a broad variety of benefits. In other words, at a cellular level you are inducing normal function; you are inducing the normal production of ATP.

However, you may be thinking about the cost. I believe it is an investment initially and it's worth it especially in the long run. What you can experience are tremendous. It is a one-time investment and it pays dividends. It pays itself off years and years to come in the future. It has a host of health benefits and it's really simple. You don't have to like change your diet; it's something that you invest in just a little bit of time on your health each day and it benefits your sleep.

For weight loss

Near infrared light therapy or photobiomodulation has been around for a few decades but it has not been used as mainstream medicine. It can be very effective for seasonal affective disorder, circadian rhythm, mismatches sleep problems various skin conditions, pain management, hair growth and accelerated wound healing

Near red light wavelengths have a specifically unique and beneficial effect on longevity.It relieves muscle pain aches and can reduce arthritis. It can promote the cover of skeletal muscle injuries, enhances physical performance and recovery time. It increases mitochondria functioning and energy levels by releasing ATP from cells and stimulating DNA/RNA synthesis.

It can boost testosterone in men, reduces inflammation, and lowers oxidative stress. It can also boost cognitive functioning by increasing the amount of mitochondria in the head. It is for better blood circulation, lymph flow vasodilation improved skin protection against wrinkles stretch marks and Sun induced aging.

Beingoverweight is something that can invite a number of other diseases like blood pressure, instability, diabetes, backache, arthritis, asthma etc. Also, being obese makes you look tall and ugly as clothes barely fit. While it is crucial to maintaining weight for the overall health of your body but at the same time it is really important that the weight loss method that you adopt is safe and has no side effects. One of such groundbreaking weight-loss technology is what is known as light therapy.

I am going to talk about near infrared and near light therapy for weight loss. How does near infrared light therapy for weight loss work?Near infrared light therapy works on a very simple mechanism which I will explain under two main points namely bioenergetics and blood flow by bioenergetics.

Near infrared light therapy simply stimulates the mitochondria and the fat cell mitochondria. When stimulated, it increases the glucose oxidation, this happens due to the fact that red lights wavelength is between 600 nanometers and 1000 nanometers, which stimulate a key copper enzyme in ourselves.Consequently,more cellular energy is produced and more glucose is burnt efficiently.This leads to less stress and healthier cells.The increasing metabolic rate ultimately leads to fat loss by blood flow.

In addition, light therapy is known to improve the blood flow in an area where it falls this makes the cells produce a large amount of energy. An improved blood flow leads to providing essential nutrients to the body making it healthy.

For fat loss & body shaping

Our bodies are directly affected by light and on how we can use this light technology to help disperse fat. It helps to trigger the fat release from the fat cells.Did you know you only have so many fat cells and that is predetermined right after you go through puberty? So it is not that we have an abundance of fat cells, it is just that our fat cells just get gorged.

What this is doing is creating lipolysis which helps to disrupt that just like breaking them down.So what is going to happen once it gets breaking down? Well your body's going to use it for energy, it is going to help shuttle it out through the lymphatics and some of it will still be retained. But which is easier?Doing the thousand crunches trying to get your abs back or melting away a little bit of the fat layer.

This is all totally healthy, effortless and it was very easy and relaxing compared to the gym.

Also, this is a safe method without any side effects unlike the other slimming procedures like surgeries and other dangerous techniques. Hence, this therapy is designed to deliver benefits without any harm to the body while safely eliminating the fat in the tissue under the skin it makes your waistline visibly less.

For Arthritis & Joint Pain

Arthritis and related joint problems can surface in over 100 different ways and affect over 50 million adults. According to the Arthritis Foundation, arthritis is actually America's top reason for disability. There are many differences on how and where arthritis develops but usually the symptoms are all the same: painful, stiff and swollen joints.

Now the treatments out there for people suffering from arthritis and joint pain are all focused on managing the disease but not actually on improving the underlying problem. These treatments range from vitamins and massage therapy to surgery and medication and they also differ in how well they work.

But sadly for most people with severe chronic arthritis the only option is to take medication for their entire lives. Nobody wants to take medication consistently throughout the course of their life. This is why many people living with arthritis are seeking out modern alternative treatments for their condition and it turns out that near red and near-infrared light therapy also called photobiomodulation or PBM for short has been studied extensively and found to provide real benefit for multiple forms of arthritis in various parts of the body.

In fact, according to these studies photobiomodulation even shows promise in physically changing the condition of the body's joints for the better.

For over a decade countless of clinical studies have supported the use of light therapy for arthritis and researchers from some of the very top medical institutions in the world have recommended it as an effective form of treatment alternative to the traditional methods including medicine.

For example, a systematic review published in the Journal of Rheumatology in the year 2000 found that light therapy provided significant results across 13 Sep clinical trials. The best results are demonstrated in people suffering from rheumatoid arthritis who reported 70 percent less pain after receiving light therapy compared to the placebo group.

In another study, in the year 2012, issued in the clinical rehabilitation participants received light therapy along with exercise they showed significant improvements for many variables including pain functionality range of motion all of this compared to the placebo treatment and it turns out that light therapy can also improve general joint problems not even related to arthritis.

Also, a 2013 systematic review in the Australian journal of physiotherapy looked at 11 clinical trials of light therapy for chronic joint disorders in the knee. The results showed that light therapy reduced joint pain while improving overall joint function.

There is strong evidence supporting the use of near red and near-infrared light therapy for reducing symptoms of arthritis and improving overall joint health.Now,these studies are just a sample of the wide body of clinical research that documents positive results when using photobiomodulation for joint pain and arthritis.

But these benefits depend on choosing a light therapy device that delivers the right wavelengths with optimal power levels for instance the Joovv light provide red and near-infrared wavelengths with professional-grade power output.

For Reversing Alzheimer's and Parkinson's diseases

As we know neurodegeneration refers to the progressive death of neurons and the two most well-known examples are Parkinson's and Alzheimer's. Over time, the symptoms get progressively worse eventually making day-to-day routine activities difficult for patients.

The current treatments for patients of both diseases offer at best symptomatic relief particularly for Parkinson's but do not provide neuroprotection or are not disease modifying at least in humans.

One of the reasons that there is so much scientific interest in near-infrared in the last few years is actually the lengthy list of conditions it appears to help with.The list extends to retinal disease, traumatic brain injury, optic nerve injury experimentally induced stroke, familiar amyotrophic lateral sclerosis which is ALSmultiple sclerosis, Parkinson's and Alzheimer's. What this has led us to believe is that these issues involve common pathways.

Now the near-infrared is proposed to work in two different ways. The first way is direct stimulation. Here, the main direct target of near-infrared appears to be cytochrome C oxidase. It is a key enzyme of the mitochondrial respiratory chain this is where the energy of the cell comes from and if energy is compromised there will be multiple issues as one could imagine. Specifically,they concluded that direct stimulation of cells with near-infrared conditions neurons to resist future damage and accelerate repair of neurons damaged by a previous or continuing insult in addition to protecting and repairing damaged or dysfunctional neurons.

There is emerging evidence from most models of traumatic brain injury that near-infrared also stimulates neurogenesis and synaptogenesis. Now with the stimulation of the neurons (creating healthy mitochondria), neurogenesis (which means new nerves coming back on track) and synaptogenesis (getting new connections of nerves), this is really quite unheard of in current medical models for Alzheimer's.

What this means is that not only does near-infrared resist and help repair damage but it also appears to help the brain create new nerve cells and new neural connections take a second to think about what this potentially means.

Finally,they talked about how these neurodegenerative diseases have been implicated as vascular disorders with suggestions that the neurodegenerative process begins with the breakdown of the integrity of small cerebral that means brain vessels and the blood-brain barrier.

Part of the neuro-protective aspect of near-infrared maybe from misses in quotations, repair of the damaged mitochondria in local endothelial cells leading subsequently to a restoration of the integrity of the endothelial network and blood-brain barrier in the region resulting ultimately an improved neuronal survival. That's the key. So direct stimulation is what the majority of the research is on and this direct stimulation seems to have absolutely incredible benefits when it comes to the problems of Alzheimer's and Parkinson's

The second way that near-infrared is proposed to work for Alzheimer's and Parkinson's is the indirect stimulation of the cells by the near-infrared so the first was the direct stimulation, this is a concept of indirect stimulation and this is a fascinating area of research and directly applies to the use of near-infrared.

There is increasing evidence that near-infrared treatment might also activate a global systemic note however while the mechanism remains unknown it presumably involves the stimulation of one or more circulating molecules or cell types possible mechanisms that they mention includes stimulation of immune cells inflammatory mediators bone marrow derived stem cells or a signaling system between mitochondria. The mechanism may not be completely understood but the point is that application of near-infrared away from the brain had a positive effect on the brain and other organs although of course less effective than the direct exposure. So what does all of this mean?

First of all, most of the results but not all are still at the proof of concept stage as the study concludes.There is much to do in further developing this treatment but the therapeutic possibilities are many and the potential outcomes very exciting so we await the outcomes of major clinical trials using near-infrared therapy on these patients with much anticipation. Hence, the recommendations that I am making here are my opinion and not necessarily the opinion of the researchers.

Direct stimulation is still and has to be at your own discretion. The research is yet to be done as to the length of exposure and the intensity of the exposure. But there are some issues with direct exposure on how will the near-infrared penetrate through the actual skull. It does penetrate but it does not penetrate particularly deep so it may have more of a help directly on Alzheimer's than it does on Parkinson's but you can read the study for more information on that. Research has shown that there is no long term side effects associated with the use of near-infrared.

So the point there is that there may be absolutely nothing to lose if the risk is high that you will be developing Alzheimer's or Parkinson's or that you have it so waiting for science to catch up has risks.Usually it takes about 10 to 15 years for research to become clinically active in other words it takes that long for research to get into the hands of most family doctors.

Note that this information is still somewhat controversial and it is still not fully clinically accepted. But it is more extremely promising than anything else in my opinion and again in conclusion this indirect use of near-infrared is probably a key component that can help so many people and there may be scenarios where people may choose at their own discretion to apply the near-infrared directly to the cranium and try to help with those scenarios through there.

For accelerated Healing

The color of red has a psychological effect of stopping traffic lights,used as stop signs and warning letters and so forth. It turns out that red light can have the potential to stop pain and inflammation.As you already know, red light is one of the component lights of white light. If you were to take white light and shine it through a crystal prism it would split into its component colors. Those component colors are from left to right: violet blue green orange yellow and so on to the right side red, science is finding that the red wavelengths have potentially therapeutic benefits.

Photobiomodulation is a property where light strikes living biological tissue and triggers a physiological response.You have heard of this phenomenon before way back into third grade. The form that you learned about is called photosynthesis. As we recall in photosynthesis, sunlight strikes the leaf of a plant where it gets absorbed by structures called chloroplasts. The chloroplasts contain chlorophyll, which is a substance that makes plants look green well, that triggers a cascade of events that essentially allow the plant to convert carbon dioxide in the air and the water into sugar. This is why plants are the source of carbohydrates.

The leading theory on how near infrared light produces photobiomodulation is via increasing cellular energy.In a typical cell, you have a membrane-nucleus little structures called mitochondria and various other supporting structures that enable the cell to respirate and perform all its functions.Now this requires energy.

Energy production happens in the structures that are called mitochondria.When red light strikes cell it gets absorbed by molecules called cytochrome C oxidase and when cytochrome C oxidase absorbs red light it increases the rate of ATP production. ATP is basically the fuel molecule of all cells.The energy stored in its bonds is what the cell uses to do things such as proliferate, regenerate, synthesize proteins, increase the metabolic rate and so forth.

The other theory is that as the cytochrome C oxidase absorbs the red light it increases the ATP production but that in turn produces more reactive oxygen species or ROS that serves to change the oxidative state of the cell which basically means it changes its electrical charge.When the oxidative state of a cell is changed, it basically up regulates genes that are associated with beneficial effects such as proliferation, increasing membrane potential, synthesizing protein and a bollock activity.All of these reactions are beneficial to wound healing and reducing inflammation.

For anti-aging

Red light therapy can improve skin clarity tone and texture, reduce fine lines wrinkles and puffy eyes, help fade skin's acne and stretch marks, enhance wound healing and circulation.

It does this simply by increasing the production of collagen and elastin. Remember that collagen is a long chain amino acid and the most abundant protein in the body. It is responsible for giving skin its elasticity; hair its strength and connective tissue its ability to hold everything in place. In fact the collagen protein makes up about 30% of the total protein in the body and 70% of the protein in the skin and now while collagen is beneficial to the entire body it's most notably beneficial to the skin.

This is because as we age the epidermic or outer layer of skin thins and loses its elasticity. As this happens, we tend to show more signs of aging and acquire more wrinkles and stretch marks but by restoring normal cellular function, because red light stimulates the production of collagen, red light therapy can help keep your skin looking healthier and younger.

Is it safe?

It sounds like this amazing thing that has a ton of health benefits and there seem to be no negative side effects. There are no side effects of photobiomodulation which is ironic because it is so much more effective than other methods like taking drugs or doing chemotherapy.

Red light therapy targets specific wavelengths of light that have the most beneficial effect on the human body it even avoids the harmful

UV rays from the Sun that in excess can be very bad for you. However, the most common side effect of red light therapy is tiredness and redness of the skin if you use it too much.

How to use near infrared and near light therapy

When it comes to red light dosage, then you have to know your devices lights power density. You can measure it at different distances with a solar power meter. In general, you can get a therapeutic benefit by exposing yourself to red light for 10 to 15 minutes while standing about 20 to 30 centimetres away from it once a day. I personally do my red light sessions in the morning or evening, in conjunction with maybe some mobility exercises, meditation lying on an acupuncture mattress or writing articles.

The ultimate guide to choosing NIR light therapy device

If you started looking at the different brands of light therapy devices there is a good chance that you may be feeling a little bit overwhelmed by the sheer number of options that are available to you.

There are major differences between the light therapy devices and there are three most critical factors to look for as you make your choice namely; the wavelengths, the intensity of the light delivered and the treatment area of the device.

Wavelengths-

Most of the devices deliver red light between 630 and 700 nanometers. You will also see devices on the market using ranges from almost orange light at 600 nanometers all the way up to 900 nanometers. You can find public studies that show the benefit of virtually all of these different wavelengths.

However the bulk of clinical research suggests that light in the mid 600 nanometer range and low to mid 1000 nanometer range is extremely effective and that's because these wavelengths have been proven to significantly enhance cellular function which ultimately results in a wide range of health benefits. Hence, it's critical to choose a device that delivers optimal wavelengths of light.

The light intensity or irradiance-

Basically this governs the amount of energy a light therapy device can deliver to your cells. Light therapy at the right wavelength can provide great benefits at relatively low intensity levels but certain benefits such as deep tissue rejuvenation require higher intensities. The problem is that a lot of companies don't even publish the intensity of their devices which makes it tough to figure out how long heat to use the product in order to receive those clinically relevant benefits. And if you get stuck with an underpowered device you have to spend a lot more time using it to get the results that you want and that actually ties into another important consideration.

The area of your body that you are planning to treat-

Most light therapy devices cover such a small treatment area that it would take 20 to 30 minutes just to treat your face and even more time if you want to treat other areas of your body. Most people simply don't have the amount of time it takes to make that work on any kind of a consistent basis. So fit it to your lifestyle. You should pick careful attention to the size of the area that you want to treat and be sure that the size of the device is applicable for that.

Generally, light therapy devices should be a device that you could use at home yet powerful enough to see quick results even for deep tissue healing and to deliver the optimal wavelengths at the proper intensity covering a large practical treatment area depending on what symptoms you're trying to treat. When you use them, you can experience the rejuvenating power of red light therapy in less than 10 minutes a day.

My experience and recommended lights for NIR light therapy

JoovvLight:

As a company they have great customer service which I am very big on. I have worked in customer service before so I am especially critical of companies. I am always watching for what is their customer service like, what is their website like, and their website is very thorough with lots of helpful information.If you are trying to figure out whether light therapy is something that is right for me, which unit do I want, they cover everything. You can email them.Call them, chat them and I have asked several questions when I was going about purchasing it and they were just super helpful and friendly, quick to respond.So, I was impressed with that and the quality of the device was awesome something.

After all my research this was a clear standout winner and the biggest thing I was looking for was EMF which is electromagnetic fields.You may have been hearing a little bit more about that.There is some concerns growing over these fields that are given off by electronic devices cell phones, TVs. I do not want to be standing in front of something every day that's harming me when it's supposed to be helping me and with the Joovvlight there are zero EMFs when you are usingit at the recommended treatment distance. So that is a big bonus right there.

Also,the quality in terms of the lifespan is great. It has a 50,000 hour life span.That is a long time fighting.So I think that I can use this for a long time without wearing it out which is also important.

And it is FDA approved. It is always nice to know about something and it is just a well-made machine. You can tell that about the machine and about the company itself they stand behind it and they are there for questions.So I have just been really impressed overall at the performance of it, how well it is made and how the company has treated me. The overall experience of it has been very positive and I am looking forward to continuing to use it.

Another thing that made me gravitate to the Joovv was that if a machine is underpowered, you are going to have to stand in front of it and use it for a lot longer.And since this machine is high quality, you can get the treatment you need and get the results you need in a quicker time so that is nice but you do still have to commit to it and stand in front of it and it is not long at all. I usually do five minutes on the front side and five minutes on the back.It can really be that quick if you want it to be and I will read a book or sometimes, I will have the TV on or I willjust stand and just kind of soak in the light.It feels very relaxing and soothing.It does not really give off any heat which is a good thing because heat can be counterproductive in certain situations.But even though there is no heat there is a certain warmth about it, just being in that light feels really good.

Another pro is that it is customizable.You can pick just red light, a combination of red and near-infrared light or just a near-infrared light. Then, they have a mini device and an original size device or a really big one; the max.And I got the combo lights and the original size so it does from the middle of my forehead to the middle of my thighs.And I am 5.10 in height, so just to kind of give you an idea of the coverage. I feel like that gets most of my body at once and I like kind of streamlining it and doing as much as possible.

So I am really happy with the size I chose and with the combination light and you can look on their website to learn more about what red light therapy offers specifically and what near-infrared light offers.

Like I wrote earlier, each of thosewavelength ranges have been proven to be effective as healing light. Why not have both, each offer different benefits and I like taking advantage of as much of those benefits as I can.Again I have just been really happy with it and it is so nice to use something and feel like your money was well spent.And I am actually experiencing tangible results from this and feeling better because I was having a lot of different stuff where it is like I am tired of this. I need to feel better, I want to feel more like myself again and I feel like this is really helping me get there so again I am excited to share it.

The cool thing about having a unit at home is that you get to use it, you and your family or your spouse or kids.And I mean have it like something that is consistently benefiting your health and the health of your family so it is very simple. All that you do is you turn the light on and you stand for period of time you feel you feel fit. So I personally do about 10-15 minutes a day and I do that within the morning or evening so that it really charges my body and charges my cells. It gets my blood flowing and my energy flowing. It is kind of if you were to sleep in a cave, a wild human as we were intended to be, and you get out of the cave in the morning in this bright Sun and you are just like whoa, just go you are like okay like that is going to wake you up. So there are few things that can really wake you up and get you going.One of them is a cold shower and the other is red light therapy. Both are awakening and they really get you going and get you charged.Keep in mind that we do generate energy from the Sun just like animals and plants and everything, our planet generates energy from the Sun as well.

All that I do is stand in front of it each day and let the light on me within about a foot or less away.So literally my face, eyes neck, chest gets this light.

If you are a male and you use this device you want the red light to hit you in your chest or on your testicles or both the reason being is because it actually boostsyour testosterone substantially as I mentioned earlier. That is great because testosterone is beneficial for many things, is going to spin for a body physique, for energy, and for sexual performance energy.This great because as men hit about 30 years old, testosterone starts to dip down this is something that keeps that going.So I and my husband stay in front of it and we literally just sit in front of it.

What most people do is they hang it on their bedroom door or maybe up their bathroom door or just on the wall like in their bedroom and they just walk up turn on the light each morning. So it is really that simple and this light is doing so much for your health and it is doing so much for your vitality.

It is definitely worth checking out and I highly encourage you to check out their website learn more and see if you can find one of their products that work for you in your home.The nice thing is there is the midlevel, so they have two of these bars. And if you want to if you areserious about your red light therapy you can get something even better, bigger and better than that probably in the next year. But they have a smaller red light therapy so if you just want to do it for your face, your skin, your wrinkles and the health of your face you can do that so they have different options.

Poly the new face of light therapy

Polyrejuve1820 LED lights emit red light energy at 633 nanometers which is proven to be among the most powerful and beneficial wavelengths. And rosacea poly is safe gentle and effective for all skin types. It is also relaxing, comforting and a great stress reliever.Poly can be used anywhere on the body.Poly is drug laser and chemically free as well as non-invasive. It requires no downtime or recovery time but makes you feel more confident, your skin will look and feel younger softer and smoother with each session.

Red light man

So how can you do some red light therapy yourself?Functional health facilities like the bulletproof labs tend to have red light beds that cost about 50 to 100 dollars for a 20-minute session or you can get yourself a red light device and you can use it at your own convenience. Or you can use a full body panel of therapeutic red and near-infrared light from a UK-based company called red light man it covers the 600 to 800 nanometer wavelength and it can be hanged on walls or the ceiling.They have several different types of devices that are smaller and can be used to target specific areas of the body as well.Red light man uses high quality LED lights and appropriate wavelengths of light with metabolic and therapeutic benefits. So, stay rejuvenated stay empowered!

Shared experiences from friends and colleagues who use near infrared and near light therapy

Here, I shared some of the reviews I got from my friends on how they feel using the near infrared light therapy. Perhaps, you will learn one or two lessons!

From Cara,

Hi Jennie,

What my experience has been like with the Joovv unit and how I am using it

First of all, I am using it for about a 10 to 12 minute use or exposure time in order to get the benefit that we are looking for from a specific Joovv unit based on its intensity and the energy.

Because it is near red light, I am trying to match my usage to the natural time of day where we would see red light meaning an hour within sunrise and an hour before sunset. So I am trying not to use it outside of those windows and don't use it midday. I do not use it before sunrise and I do not use it after dark. I do not know if there is any research that says I should not use it outside of sunrise and sunset but like I said, I am just trying to match my increased red light exposure to the natural times of day. It is really important to me that we try to match and optimize our circadian rhythm so I am really paying close attention to my exposure to light and how it impacts my health, my sleep cycles and my biological clock.

The other thing that I do for photo bio modulation is I use the human charger.It is great for jet lag but I loved it during the winter months when we move into daylight savings time.So from November to March when we spring forward again with our clocks, I use the human charger for about 10 to 15 minutes before sunset.The reason I do this is that when the Sun goes down early, let's say it goes down at 5 pm, I would start to feel sleepy around 8 pm and if I don't go to bed right then I am secreting extra cortisol to kind of get a second wind and stay awake until I may go to bed at9:30, 10:30, or 11 o'clock. So what I will do is I use the human charger right before sunset to give myself a non-caffeine energy boost and it will trick my body into thinking that it's not quite time to wind down.then what I've noticed is that I will start to wind down a little bit later than when I don't use it.So somewhere in that 9, 9:30 or 10 o'clock range then I can fall asleep without having to have had that cortisol boost which we don't want.If you know about the cortisol cycle we want it to be at its lowest right before we go to bed so we do not want that little secondary peak between 8 p.m. and 10 p.m. and that's something that I've noticed and it made a big difference for me I don't have science behind that it's just personal experience.

Thank you.

From Victoria.

Hi Jennie,

So again, I am using the light in the morning within 30 minutes of waking up. It is part of my morning routine. There are some days where I honestly do not feel like doing it as the first thing in the morning, so I will do it at night. I believe my morning routine should be something that sets me up for success for any given day. It is not something that I have to follow like a checklist as if skipping it on that thing is going to make me less of a person on that day. And I caution everyone against falling in love or being "married" to that morning routine as if it is something that holds power outside of you. Like I said, if I do not feel like doing it I do not most of the time. I do it first thing in the morning if I do not, I get it done at night sometime around sunset. My experience is it definitely warms me up. I can feel it right now as I write this. I am actually sweating a little bit and I am not even as close to it as I normally am. I am about a foot and a half maybe two feet away from it right now. I can feel the warmth and the heat from it which is interesting because it is not really designed to be a heat source like a sauna but it does provide its energy.These are energy waves and they will warm you up.

So honestly, I do feel somewhat energized. I feel sort of like a clean boost but it is not something like drinking coffee and you feel that kind of energy.It is one of those things as you heard that the more you use it the more the effects.When I use it I feel warmer and I feel sort of energized.But I feel energized at the cellular level, it feels like a real boost and I feel it especially in the morning.If I do it first thing in the morning I feel that boost, I feel awake and alive. Thank you.

From Whitten M.

Hi Jennie J. Martins,

Joovv veterans of light is near red and infrared light

You can get light therapy up different places but I really wanted one that I can use at home because I have a one-year-old and to get him to sit in front of anywhere for a period of time it is kind of difficult and as much as I wanted to do it with him twice a day every day going somewhere is just not realistic whatsoever.So I am looking into the different devices they can have at home you just have to be careful what specific wavelengths they deliver.

After tons and tons and tons of research the Joovv Light ended up getting the mini combo device which is a mixture of 50% red and 50% and infra-red and honestly I have been loving it for multiple reasons.

You can go to their website because they have a bunch of amazing information and they provide you with all the scientific studies that have been done on red and near-infrared light. So it is doing something good for yourself.

When I was writing this mail, I was standing in front of my red light device and I felt the rejuvenating effect on my skin.Another one of those advantages of working at home is that you get to do red light therapy conveniently. Thank you.

So let me hear what you think. If you have used neared and near infrared light therapy, post on comment section.Share and buy this book with the people in your life who you know will benefit from and enjoy the things that I have been talking about here.

Frequently Asked Questions on NIR and red light therapy

Below are randomly selected interview questions and answers from health experts and users of the near infrared light therapy.

What is photobiomodulation and what are the wavelengths that we need to be focused on now?

So there are specific wavelengths that have been documented to have the most profound effect on enhancing cellular function and the wavelengths that are supported by the research are in the red and near-infrared spectrum and what is called the therapeutic window and the reason that this range of wavelengths is so important is they have the unique ability to penetrate human tissue compared to other wavelengths of the light spectrum. They have ability to do this.

So wavelengths that are longer than 1000 nanometers for example are very quickly absorbed by the moisture in our tissue and so the resulting effect is the radiant heat and so they are not able to penetrate to deeper tissue the same way. So the specific wavelengths that are in the mid 600 at 660 nanometers as well as 850 nanometers which is in the near infrared spectrum.

What's really going on when we stand in front of these red lights?

There are some different theories as to the mechanism of action for photobiomodulation but probably the most respected theory is this concept of activating an enzyme called cytochrome C oxidase or C co.

Sometimes,you will see the acronym C co used in clinical research but during the fourth phase of cellular respiration that enzyme went under stress will bind to nitric oxide which prevents the production of ATP synthase which is a precursor to ATP.So what specific wavelengths within that therapeutic window do is they actually break that bond between cytochrome C oxidase and nitric oxide almost releasing it to help induce normal cellular function during that fourth phase of respiration. That is probably the most respected theory.There is also other things going on like enhanced gene transcription because of our OS signaling during a light therapy. That is another sort of theory as to what is going on at a cellular level but the activation of cytochrome C oxidase is at the core of what what's going on with photobiomodulation.

Is that the single thing that leads to this kind of impressive list of benefits from light therapy?

Yesabsolutely, why you get such a broad variety of benefits is because at a cellular level you are inducing normal function, you are inducing the normal production of ATP which is the energy currency of our cells

From the list of benefits it is likely that most people are skeptical like there is no way that light can do this type of this type of thing?

All of those benefits are documented in peer-reviewed clinical studies. So it is hard to argue when you see thousands of thousands of studies that are supporting these types of benefits.So the evidence is there but rightfully I can imagine that some people are pretty skeptical.

Describe photobiomodulation?

The easy way I like to describe that to people in a way they can visualize is if you are outside on a hot sunny day and you feel that intense sunlight and then a cloud goes over you immediately. You will notice that it is like somebody flipped a switch and the heat you were feeling in your body is suddenly cut way down.The visible light and the UV spectrum is affected very little by those clouds but you notice the far infrared those wavelengths have been for the vast majority of that energy has been absorbed by the moisture in the cloud.

Saunas versus photobiomodulation?

They are just two distinct therapies and their mechanism of action are distinctly different. You cannot have a device that does both. They are different.So a heat lamp thatis decent for generating heat for the purpose of saunasis poor for the purpose of photobiomodulation, because they are really inefficient heat and not optimal. So they are two distinct therapiesand both have been documented clinically to work well just different concepts.

What is the best practices with light therapy device?

The best practices really come down to how you can implement it as part of your daily routine.So as with any photobiomodulation therapy is something ideally that you do daily.I do have people that do it multiple times a day but it is definitely something that takes that consistency. Is critical to seeing the long-term benefits while you certainly can have reduction in pain or inflammation from a single treatment for overall cellular function you're definitely better off to have a daily or consistent treatment.

I noticed right away when I plugged it in turned it on about half the lights were not on?

The ones that you cannot see are the ones that are not in the visible spectrum so they are actually on you just cannot see them.

How are you guys using it on a daily basis?

Fundamentally trying to fit it into your daily routine isoptimal and so I personally use it in the morning just because that tendsto fit well into my daily routine.Now if I am trying to treat something specifically, if I have got some torn up hands hamstrings or I tweaked my knee or something, I may try to fit in a secondary treatment towards the end of the day.But typically I use it in the morning or you can target specific areas more than just like a daily full-body treatment.

How to use it either for prophylactic reasons or proactive health?

Use at a distance of about six inches away from your device whether standing or sitting and gofor about eight to ten minutes. Somedevices at that distance will deliver about six joules of energy.So a 10 minute treatment is going to receive about 60 joules of energy which is clinically significant.But if you have got something specific that you are trying to treat, fitting in another session is probably ideal versus going really long in one session.That is probably clinically a little bit superior to just a really prolonged session.So that is why I probably recommend splitting those up.If you are going to do multiple sessions per day, it is perfect. I tend to do treatments more in the evening. I found that it relaxes me and helps me sleep better. I kind of recover from the stress of the day. But if it is a cloudy or rainy day I definitely enjoy a morning session. So it depends on what is going on that day but I would tend to do more evening treatments.It really depend on your own personal preference, what fits in your schedule and what you personally enjoy.You bring an element of bio-hacking to it because if you understand light, when you need light and how it works, you can use it at different times for different things on different days.

The morning or evening session is probably ideal because it mimics the natural sunrise and sunset.But you can still use in in the midday if that is the best time for you. However, to optimize the performance morning and or evening is probably ideal.

Where do you see the future of this going that you can talk about now?

I was fascinated by how much clinical data there is with respect to photobiomodulation. Why does it seem like there's still a lack of awareness despite the overabundance of clinical data?

I think we are getting there and within the next five to ten years there will be a significant percentage of the population that has a light therapy device in their own home just because the evidence is too hard to ignore.And so I do think at over time if we do a good job to continue to educate the marketplace on the concept of how our bodies metabolize light it will become a lot more a lot more prevalent.

Top three tips to live optimal?

I would say **tip number one** would be you can try to get a healthy dose of natural sunlight in the morning primarily to reset your circadian rhythm. I will go with the amazing benefits from the Earth's gravitational field.So it is most people are aware of grounding but if you haven't heard of the concept of the Earth's magnetic field and its

.mpact on your cellular function definitely look into that it's pretty .ncredible.

Second tip - I think fasting

There's obviously been a fair amount of education recently around fasting. Dr. R. Patrick has done a great job at Devaney. I have practiced or tried to practice as I can intermittent fasting. Sometimes it is difficult with kids but try to squeeze in that feeding window within six hours but I personally want to toy around more with like prolongedfast either on a monthly or quarterly basis. I have heard Ferris mention that several times and another kind of other folks I practice prolonged fasting right now and so that is something that I personally kind of want to play more often.We will follow up on that one with you.

How do you view the eating window you mentioned?

Like trying to keep it to six hours but right yes I mean so like on a pragmatic basis what that looks like for me personally is typically I will have my first meal of the day usually around one o'clock or so and then try to eat by 6:00 or finish up like a dinner by it.So it is usually just two meals right at dinner like six or seven sometimes. There is some I will snack a little bit try to as healthy as possible in between the two. I mean if you are consuming butter or something that is a macronutrient. I think that probably interrupts the fasting window and I look at my windows I don't really worry about how long it is on any given day.It is just some days.I may be at a conference and I might get a snack because I am starving and then I may not eat again until I leave the conference. So maybe on such days, my window is eight hours maybe at home it is two hours one day and then the next day it is four or six.But it is flexible and my goal on any given day is to keep it as small as possible.

Tip number three

Tryto practice gratitude more consistently.Practicing even simple gratitude on a daily basis and allowing that to sort of reset your mind.

Tip number four

Look for ways to reduce stress on your body.Most of us have heard about the dangers of EMS for example, take a stock around you, what are some things that you can do to avoid the clear hazards that have been identified.

Whether it is a cell phone, carrying that in your body clearly is not a good idea, put that in airplane mode.When you have to have it on you, set it a little bit of ways from you so you are not exposing yourself to those dangers of Wi-Fi.Clearly that is something you can turn off at night.With simple tips like that you can really reduce some of the hazards and stressors that you are putting on your body and cells on a daily basis.

CONCLUSION

Red light therapy as a healing technology delivers energy to cells by applying a range of visible and invisible wavelengths of light.

Other names for red light therapy include low-level laser therapy,photonic stimulation, phototherapy, biostimulation bios, low intensity light therapy, photobiomodulation, photobiostimulation, etc.

Red light therapy has been proven effective for a wide range of conditions including pain relief, increasing bone density, preventing hair loss, cognitive enhancement, fat reduction, wound healing, increase testosterone, for hairgrowth reducing anxiety and depression, smoking cessation, building muscle, healing acne, anti-aging, and many more indications

This book is as much about near infrared light therapy and red light therapy.Near infrared light is another form of electromagnetic radiation and is similar to red light in both frequency as well as biological effects.

Near infrared and red light therapies have virtually no adverse side effects. However, they have a mountainof evidence supporting their remarking therapeutic value.

ABOUT THE AUTHOR

Jennie J. Martins brings you the message of near infra and near light therapy as a powerful tool to heal your body and optimize your health. As a health expert, she writes to throw more light around this topic- Near infrared and near light therapy. She has benefitted immensely from near light therapy and she shares her experiences with you. Hence, she takes you through the science of how to use near-infrared and red light therapy to improve your health and your life in dozens of ways.

Printed in Great Britain
by Amazon

67120890R00075